Tabl

Vegan Air Fryer Cookbook

40 Tasty Vegan Air Fryer Recipes

Cheesy Potato Squares

Tasty and healthy potatoes with the unique flavor of garlic, almonds, and paprika. Excellent choice to enjoy with your family!

Serving Size: 4 persons

Prep Time: 5 minutes

Cooking Time: 20 minutes

Ingredients Needed

- 1 pound of potatoes
- 1 Tbsp. of olive oil
- 1 teaspoon of sea salt
- 1 teaspoon of pepper
- 1 teaspoon of garlic powder
- ¾ cup of almonds
- 1 teaspoon of paprika
- Juice from 1 lemon
- ¾ cup of water
- Salt and pepper to taste

Method of Preparation

- Preheat the air fryer to 375°F for about 5 minutes.
- Wash the potatoes and then cut them in large squares. Put them into a large bowl.
- Mix the olive oil, salt, pepper and garlic powder.
- Add the oil, salt, pepper, and garlic powder to the potatoes.
- Spread this mixture over all the potatoes. Put the potatoes on the air fryer and cook for 20 minutes, stirring every 2-3 minutes until golden.
- In a blender, mix the almonds, paprika and lemon. Blend and add water as needed until you get a "cheesy" consistency.

- Pour this mixture over the potatoes and cook for 3 more minute.
- Serve and enjoy!

Nutritional Analysis (Per Serving)
Calories 219
Total fat 12.7g
Carbs 23g
Protein 6g

Sweet Potato fingers

A delicious and sweet snack you can have any time of the day!

Serving Size: 4 persons

Prep Time: 20 minutes

Cooking Time: 30 minutes

Ingredients Needed

- 2 medium sweet potatoes
- 1 tablespoon of cornstarch
- 1/4 teaspoon of garlic powder
- 1/2 teaspoon of sea salt
- ½ cup of ketchup
- 2 tablespoon of olive oil or coconut oil

Method of Preparation

- Boil a pot with water and add the sweet potatoes into it for about 10 minutes or until ready.
- Remove them from the pot and remove the skin from the sweet potatoes.
- Grate the potatoes with a grater.
- Place the grated sweet potatoes into a bowl and mix it with the cornstarch, garlic powder, and sea salt.
- Shape this mixture into medium cylinders of the size of your thumb.
- Turn on the air fryer to 375 F.
- Coat the fryer with the olive oil.
- Cook the sweet potato fingers for 15-20 minutes, stirring frequently until browned.
- Serve and enjoy with ketchup!

Nutritional Analysis (Per Serving)
Calories 186
Total fat 7.2g
Carbs 30.4g
Protein 1.7g

Air Fried Sesame Zucchini

Amazing chicken with the inspiring taste of sesame seeds!
Serving Size: 4 persons
Prep Time: 20 minutes
Cooking Time: 20 minutes
Ingredients Needed

- 2 pounds of Zucchini
- ½ cup of cornstarch
- ½ teaspoon of sea salt
- ½ teaspoon of white pepper
- ⅛ cup of soy sauce
- ⅛ cup of ketchup
- 1 tablespoon of sugar
- 1 tablespoon of apple cider vinegar
- 2 tablespoon of coconut oil
- 1 chipotle chili
- 20 gr of ginger
- 3 garlic cloves
- ½ onion
- 1 tablespoon of sesame seeds

Method of Preparation

- Mix the cornstarch, salt, and pepper.
- Cut the zucchini's in half, lengthwise and add them into the bowl with the cornstarch mixture. Coat them well.
- Preheat the air fryer to 375F for 3 minutes.
- Add the coconut oil into the air fryer and cook the zucchini for 5-7 minutes on each side.
- In a pan, toast the sesame seeds for about 2 minutes until

lightly browned.
- Thinly chop the ginger, chipotle, garlic and onion.
- In a bowl, mix the soy sauce, ketchup, sugar, apple cider vinegar, chipotle, onion, garlic, ginger and sesame seeds.
- Heat a pan and pour that mixture over it. Remove zucchini from the fryer and add them to the sauce. Cook for 3-4 minutes. Serve and sprinkle some sesame seeds over it. Enjoy!

Nutritional Analysis (Per Serving)
Calories 316
Total fat 26.8g
Carbs 20.6g
Protein 9.3g

Doughnuts

Interesting, delicious and easy way to eat some tasty doughnuts using your air fryer~

Serving Size: 8 persons

Prep Time: 100 minutes

Cooking Time: 30 minutes

Ingredients Needed

- 1/4 cup of warm water
- 2 tablespoon of sugar
- 1 teaspoon of dry yeast
- 8 ounces of flour
- 1/4 teaspoon of sea salt
- 1/4 cup of soy milk
- ½ stick of butter
- 1 large egg
- 4 ounces of powdered sugar
- 1 cup of water

Method of Preparation

- In a bowl, mix the warm water, yeast and ½ tablespoon of sugar and let that mixture stand for about 5 minutes.
- Melt the butter.
- In a different bowl, mix the flour, salt, and remaining sugar. Add to this mixture the soy milk, butter, and egg. Mix until you have a soft dough.
- Place the dough into a greased bowl and cover it with a plastic paper. Let it grow until its size doubles for about an hour.
- Place this dough onto a floured surface and roll this dough to ¼ inches.

- With a doughnut cutter, cut the dough and set aside all the uncooked doughnuts. Gathered all the dough leftovers and repeat this step over and over again.
- Let the uncooked doughnuts grow for about 30 minutes.
- Turn on an air fryer to 350 F.
- Place uncooked doughnuts over an air fryer basket and cook until browned for about 4 or 5 minutes. Repeat the process until everything is cooked.
- In a bowl, mix the powdered sugar and water.
- Deep the doughnut into this mixture.
- Serve and enjoy!

Nutritional Analysis (Per Serving)
Calories 234
Total fat 6.8g
Carbs 39.4 g
Protein 4.2g

Pecan Banana Bread

A sweet and tender taste to enjoy with a delicious cup of coffee. The pecans really give this desert something special!

Serving Size: 8 persons

Prep Time: 20 minutes

Cooking Time: 30 minutes

Ingredients Needed

- 3 ounces of whole wheat flour
- ½ tablespoon of cinnamon
- 2 large bananas
- 1 teaspoon of sea salt
- ½ teaspoon of baking soda
- 3 tablespoons of sugar
- 2 eggs
- ½ cup of yogurt
- 3 tablespoon coconut oil
- ⅛ cup of vanilla extract
- 2 ounces of pecan nuts
- Coconut oil to grease

Method of Preparation

- Grease a 6 inch round cake pan with coconut oil.
- Mash the bananas.
- In a bowl, mix the flour, cinnamon, salt, and baking soda.
- In a different bowl, mix the eggs, mashed bananas, yogurt, sugar, coconut oil, and vanilla extract.
- Gently mix both the banana mixture and the flour mixture.
- Add the pecan nuts into the baking pan.
- Place the previous mixture into the round cake pan with the

pecans.

- Heat the air fryer to 350 F and place the pan into the fryer and let it cook for 25-30 minutes.
- Let it cool for 20 minutes and then turn over the pan to remove the round cake.
- Serve and enjoy!

Nutritional Analysis (Per Serving)
Calories 208
Total fat 11.7g
Carbs 23g
Protein 4.5g

Crunchy Avocado Fries

Creamy and crunchy fried avocado slices that will make you long for more! Enjoy!

Serving Size: 4 persons

Prep Time: 10 minutes

Cooking Time: 15 minutes

Ingredients Needed

- 2 ounces of flour
- 1 teaspoon of pepper
- ⅛ cup of water
- 1 cup of panko
- 2 large avocados
- 2 tablespoons of coconut oil
- 1 teaspoon of sea salt
- 1/4 cup of Caesar dressing
- 1 lemon

Method of Preparation

- Cut the avocados in half, remove the seeds and cut them into wedges. Put them in a bowl and sprinkle lemon juice over them to prevent them from turning black.
- In a different bowl mix the pepper, salt, and panko. Add water if the mixture is too thick.
- Heat the air fryer to 375 F.
- Deep each avocado wedge into the panko mixture.
- Place the avocado wedges into the fryer until browned for about 5 minutes.
- Serve with Caesar dressing and enjoy!

Nutritional Analysis (Per Serving)
Calories 334
Total fat 26.3g
Carbs 43g
Protein 10.3g

Air Fryer Garlicky Plantain

Amazing meatballs with the super tasty garlic flavor that will make you crave for more

Serving Size: 10 persons

Prep Time: 15 minutes

Cooking Time: 15 minutes

Ingredients Needed

- 2 tablespoons of coconut oil
- 1 small onion
- 5 cloves of garlic
- ¼ cup of panko
- ⅛ cup of almond milk
- 1 pound of plantains
- 1 parsley sprig
- ½ tablespoon of rosemary leaves
- ½ tablespoon of thyme leaves
- ½ teaspoon of sea salt

Method of Preparation

- Thinly chop the onion, garlic, parsley, rosemary, and thyme and put them in a bowl.
- Cut the plantains into 4 parts.
- Mix the onion mixture and add the panko, sea salt, and the milk.
- Coat the plantain parts with that mixture and set them apart.
- Turn on the air fryer to 375 F.
- Place the plantains into the air fryer and cook for 10-12 minutes.
- Serve and enjoy!

Nutritional Analysis (Per Serving)
Calories 169
Total fat 9.4g
Carbs 3.4g
Protein 7.1g

Avocado Wraps

Tasty and creamy avocado wraps with a refreshing taste of tomato and basil!

Serving Size: 4 persons
Prep Time: 15 minutes
Cooking Time: 20 minutes

Ingredients Needed

- 3 large avocados
- 8 egg roll wrappers
- 1 large tomato
- 1 pinch of sea salt
- 1 pinch of white pepper
- 1 tablespoon of coconut oil
- 1 sprig of basil
- ½ onion
- ½ cup of water
- 1 small capsicum

Method of Preparation

- Thinly slice the tomato, onion, basil, and capsicum (remove the seeds).
- Mash the avocados.
- Heat a pan with ½ tbsp. of coconut oil and add the chopped ingredients along with the water. Let it cook for 5 minutes, stir constantly until you form a sauce consistency. Add salt and pepper.
- Place the egg roll wrappers on a flat surface and distribute them on each wrapper tomato sauce and avocado.
- Wrap the wrapper and with a brush with water seal the

wrappers.

- Preheat air fryer to 375 F and put the remaining coconut oil into it.
- Place the wrappers into the fryer and let them cook for about 5 minutes until golden.
- Serve and enjoy!

Nutritional Analysis (Per Serving)
Calories 449
Total fat 24.5
Carbs 51.8g
Protein 9.5g

Oregano Air Fried Ravioli

A delicious and sweet snack you can have any time of the day!

Serving Size: 4 persons

Prep Time: 5 minutes

Cooking Time: 25 minutes

Ingredients Needed

- 1 Sprig of fresh oregano
- 1 Sprig of fresh basil
- 1 cup of chickpeas, cooked
- ½ pound of vegan ravioli
- 1 tablespoon of coconut oil
- 2 cloves of garlic
- Salt and pepper to taste
- Cooking spray
- 1 ounce of sesame seeds

Method of Preparation

- Thinly chopped the basil, oregano, and garlic.
- Heat a pan with coconut oil and cook the chickpeas, basil, oregano, and garlic. Cook for 2-3 minutes.
- Heat air fryer to 375 F.
- Stuff each ravioli with chickpeas mixture. Seal each ravioli with water.
- Place ravioli into the air fryer and sprinkle sesame seeds over them. Cook for 8-10 minutes until golden.
- Serve and enjoy!

Nutritional Analysis (Per Serving)

Calories 283

Total fat 10.2g
Carbs 38.3g
Protein 11.9g

Vegan Air Fryer Quesadillas

Delicious quesadillas made with cashews and almonds!
Serving Size: 4 persons
Prep Time: 15 minutes
Cooking Time: 25 minutes
Ingredients Needed

- ¼ cup of cashews
- ¼ cup of slivered almonds
- 2 tablespoons of cornstarch
- 1 teaspoon of apple cider vinegar
- 1 cup of water
- 4 wheat tortillas (8 inches)
- 1 tablespoon of coconut oil
- Salt and pepper to taste
- ¼ cup of basil leaves

Method of Preparation

- Heat a pot with 1 cup of water and put the cashews and almond into it and let them boil for 5 minutes. Let it cool. Add the cornstarch and stir until there are no lumps.
- Add the vinegar. Season with salt and pepper.
- Place this mixture into a blender, and blend until smooth.
- Heat this mixture again for about 3 minutes until you have a "cheesy" consistency.
- Chop the basil leaves.
- Take the wheat tortillas and distribute the cashew mixture over them and fold them in half.
- Heat air fryer to 375 F.
- Place the quesadillas into the fryer and cook for 10-12 minutes

until golden.
- Serve with basil leaves and enjoy!

Nutritional Analysis (Per Serving)
Calories 299
Total fat 14.3g
Carbs 34.8g
Protein 7.6g

Air Fryer Coconut Potato Chips

A nice, simple and healthy way to enjoy some crunchy potato chips!
Serving Size: 4 persons
Prep Time: 5 minutes
Cooking Time: 12 minute
Ingredients Needed

- 1 pound of russet potatoes
- 2 tablespoon of coconut oil
- 2 tablespoon of cilantro leaves
- 1 clove of garlic
- 1 pinch of sea salt
- 1 pinch of black pepper

Method of Preparation

- Thinly slice the potatoes and put the slices into a bowl with water.
- Thinly chop the cilantro leaves and garlic.
- Heat air fryer to 375 F.
- Coat the potato chips with coconut oil.
- Place the chips into the air fryer and add the garlic and cilantro.
- Cook for 10-15 minutes until golden.
- Serve and enjoy!

Nutritional Analysis (Per Serving)
Calories 138
Total fat 6.9g
Carbs 18.1g

Protein 2g

California Air Fryer Rolls

Delicious Sushi rolls with avocado, carrot, and cucumber!

Serving Size: 4 persons

Prep Time: 10 minutes

Cooking Time: 20 minutes

Ingredients Needed

- 3 Sheets of nori
- ½ pound of sushi rice, cooked
- ½ cucumber
- ½ carrot
- 2 medium avocados
- ¼ cup of soy sauce
- 2 ounces of sesame seeds
- ¼ cups of panko
- ¼ cup of water
- Salt and pepper

Method of Preparation

- Cut the carrot and cucumber into juliennes.
- Cut the avocados in half, remove the seeds and slice them up.
- Put a nori sheet on a makiso and put some rice over the sheet.
- In the middle of the nori, put some cucumber, carrot and avocado slices. Add salt and pepper and sesame seeds.
- Wrap the nori to form a sushi roll.
- Brush with water each roll and coat them with panko.
- Heat an air fryer to 375 F.
- Place California rolls in the fryer and cook for 8-10 minutes.
- Serve with soy sauce, enjoy!

Nutritional Analysis (Per Serving)
Calories 484
Total fat 21.2g
Carbs 64.3g
Protein 5.3g

Cauliflower and Avocado Tacos

Delicious Mexican food to enjoy in a healthy way!

Serving Size: 4 persons

Prep Time: 10 minutes

Cooking Time: 15 minutes

Ingredients Needed

- 1 Large avocado
- 1 Large Cauliflower
- 1 cup of cherry tomatoes
- 1 chipotle chili
- ½ onion
- 2 tablespoons of coconut oil
- 1 tablespoon of complete seasoning
- 8 small corn tortillas
- ½ cabbage
- Salt and pepper

Method of Preparation

- In a stove, boil some water and add the chipotle, cherry tomatoes and half onion. Boil for 5 minutes. Add salt and pepper.
- Blend the previous mixture in a blender until smooth.
- Cut the cauliflower into small florets.
- Shred the cabbage.
- Cut the avocado in half, remove the seed and slice it.
- Mix the cabbage and cauliflower in a bowl and add complete seasoning, salt, and pepper.
- Heat air fryer to 375 F.
- Add the coconut oil into the fryer and add the cauliflower

mixture. Let it cook for 15 minutes, stir constantly.

- Place tortillas on a flat surface and put cauliflower mixture on each tortilla and top with avocado and chipotle sauce. Enjoy!

Nutritional Analysis (Per Serving)
Calories 219
Total fat 17.1g
Carbs 16.7g
Protein 4.3g

Broccoli Potato "meatballs"

Delicious potato balls with kale garlic and almond milk!

Serving Size: 4 persons

Prep Time: 20 minutes

Cooking Time: 20 minutes

Ingredients Needed

- 2 large potatoes
- 1 tablespoon of coconut oil
- 2 cloves of garlic
- 4 cups of broccoli florets
- ⅛ cup of soy milk
- ¼ teaspoon of kosher salt
- ¼ teaspoon of white pepper

Method of Preparation

- Peel the potatoes.
- Cut the potatoes into four parts.
- Boil a pot with 2 cups of water and place the potatoes into the pot. Let them boil for 8 minutes until they are soft.
- Thinly chop the garlic and broccoli.
- In a bowl, mash the potatoes. Add the garlic, broccoli, milk, salt, and pepper and mix well.
- Form 2 inches balls with the mashed potatoes and put them in a bowl. Cover the bowl with plastic wrap and refrigerate for 30 min.
- Heat your air fryer to 375 F and add coconut oil to it.
- Place the "meatballs" in the fryer and cook for 12 min until golden.
- Serve and enjoy!

Nutritional Analysis (Per Serving)
Calories 223
Total fat 5g
Carbs 40g
Protein 7.4g

Cilantro Air Fryer Falafel

Tasty falafel made from chickpeas, cilantro and the inspiring taste of garlic!

Serving Size: 4 persons

Prep Time: 10 minutes

Cooking Time: 20 minutes

Ingredients Needed

- 1 ½ cups of chickpeas, soaked
- 1 cup of cilantro leaves
- 1 tablespoon of olive oil
- ½ onion
- 1 head of garlic
- 2 tablespoon of flour
- 1 teaspoon of sea salt
- 1 teaspoon of pepper
- 1 teaspoon of complete seasoning
- 1 tablespoon of basil

Method of Preparation

- Boil the chickpeas with 2 cups of water for 2 minutes.
- Thinly chop the cilantro leaves, onion, garlic, and basil.
- In a food processor, blend the chickpeas with olive oil, sea salt, and pepper for 1 minute.
- Mix the chickpeas with the chopped ingredients.
- Place this mixture in the freezer for 10 minutes.
- Remove from the freezer and for 3 inches patties with the mixture.
- Coat the patties with the flour.
- Heat air fryer to 375 F.

- Place the patties into the fryer and cook for 10 minutes until browned.
- Serve and enjoy!

Nutritional Analysis (Per Serving)
Calories 326
Total fat 8.1g
Carbs 50.5g
Protein 15.2g

Vegan Air Fryer Thai Bites

Tasty bites made from carrots, broccoli, and cauliflower!

Serving Size: 6 persons

Prep Time: 20 minutes

Cooking Time: 30 minutes

Ingredients Needed

- 3 cups of broccoli florets
- 3 cups of cauliflower florets
- 4 large carrots
- 1 Red onion
- 3 leeks
- 1 cup of coconut milk
- 3 tablespoon of flour
- 1 tablespoon of chopped fresh ginger
- 3 cloves of garlic
- 1 tablespoon of curry paste
- 1 tablespoon of cilantro leaves
- 1 tablespoon of complete seasoning
- Salt and pepper to taste
- 2 tablespoons of coconut oil

Method of Preparation

- Thinly chop the broccoli, cauliflower, carrot, onion, leeks, garlic, and cilantro leaves.
- Heat a pan with 1 tablespoon of coconut oil and cook the chopped vegetables for about 5 minutes, stirring constantly. Add the curry paste and ginger and continue stirring until the onion is transparent.
- Add the coconut milk, complete seasoning, and flour and

allow simmering for 10 minutes, until you have a paste consistency.

- Place mixture in a medium Pyrex and cover it with plastic wrap. Refrigerate for 30 minutes.
- Heat air fryer to 375 F.
- Remove Pyrex from the fridge and cut the mixture into medium squares.
- Place squares in the fryer and cook for 10 minutes.
- Serve and enjoy!

Nutritional Analysis (Per Serving)
Calories 250
Total fat 16g
Carbs 25.5g
Protein 5.3g

Garlic and Lemon Roasted Chickpeas

Delicious chickpeas with a citric taste of lemon and garlic!

Serving Size: 4 persons

Prep Time: 5 minutes

Cooking Time: 20 minutes

Ingredients Needed

- 2 cups of chickpeas, soaked
- 1 tablespoon of coconut oil
- 2 medium lemons
- 3 garlic cloves
- 1 tablespoon of dried oregano
- 1 tablespoon of dried basil
- 1 tablespoon of dried thyme
- ½ teaspoon of sea salt
- ½ teaspoon of black pepper

Method of Preparation

- Grate the zest of the lemons.
- Extract the juice from the lemons.
- Thinly chop the garlic, oregano, basil, and thyme.
- In a bowl, mix all of the ingredients together until well combined.
- Heat air fryer to 375 F.
- Place mixture into the air fryer and cook for 25 minutes. Stir the mixture after 12 minutes.
- Serve and enjoy!

Nutritional Analysis (Per Serving)

Calories 411

Total fat 9.7g
Carbs 65.4g
Protein 11.5g

Airfryer Cauliflower Bowl

Delicious cauliflower with a taste of garlic, onion, and mushrooms!
Serving Size: 4 persons
Prep Time: 5 minutes
Cooking Time: 25 minutes
Ingredients Needed

- 1 large cauliflower
- 1 large onion
- 6 cloves of garlic
- 2 tablespoon of soy sauce
- 1 tablespoon of apple cider vinegar
- 1 tablespoon of coconut oil
- ½ tablespoon of brown sugar
- 2 scallions
- 2 cups of sliced mushrooms

Method of Preparation

- Cut the cauliflower into bite-size florets.
- Cut the onion into large squares.
- Thinly chop the garlic.
- Slice the scallions.
- Heat air fryer to 375 F.
- In a bowl, mix the soy sauce, vinegar, and sugar.
- Put the coconut oil into the fryer and then add the cauliflower florets. Cook for 10 minutes and then add soy sauce mixture, mushrooms, onion, and scallions. Cook for 5-7 more minutes.
- Serve in a bowl and enjoy!

Nutritional Analysis (Per Serving)

Calories 123
Total fat 3.8g
Carbs 19.6g
Protein 6.6g

Sweet Potato French Fries

Crunchy and sweet! This sweet potato French fries have a remarkable flavor of thyme!

Serving Size: 4 persons

Prep Time: 5 minutes

Cooking Time: 20 minutes

Ingredients Needed

- 2 large sweet potatoes
- 1 sprig of thyme
- 2 tablespoons of coconut oil
- 1 teaspoon of complete seasoning
- ½ teaspoon of Himalayan salt
- ½ teaspoon of black pepper

Method of Preparation

- Wash the sweet potatoes.
- Cut the potatoes in half wide wise and then cut them into juliennes.
- Put the slices in a bowl with water.
- Remove the thyme leaves from the sprig and thinly chop them.
- Mix the chopped thyme with the salt, pepper, and complete seasoning.
- Heat air fryer to 375 F.
- Put the coconut oil into the fryer. Add the sweet potatoes into the fryer and pour the seasoning over them. Cook for 20/25 minutes, depending on how crunchy you want your potatoes.
- Serve and enjoy!

Nutritional Analysis (Per Serving)

Calories 141
Total fat 7g
Carbs 19.6
Protein 1.1g

Spinach Air Fryer Breakfast Burritos

Tasty and amazing burrito, made with peanut butter, spinach and potatoes!

Serving Size: 4 persons
Prep Time: 20 minutes
Cooking Time: 30 minutes

Ingredients Needed

- 4 large wheat tortillas
- 2 tablespoons of peanut butter
- 1 cup of broccoli florets
- 1 cup of spinach leaves
- 1 tablespoon of coconut oil
- 1 large russet potato
- ½ cup of water
- ½ teaspoon of sea salt
- ½ teaspoon of pepper

Method of Preparation

- Peel the potato.
- Cut the potato into large squares.
- Boil the potato with 2 cups of water for 5 minutes until it is soft.
- Chop the broccoli.
- Heat a pan with ½ tbsp. of coconut oil and cook the broccoli and the spinach for 3-4 minutes.
- Mash the potato.
- In a bowl, mix the mashed potato with the peanut butter, broccoli, and spinach. Mix in the salt and pepper.
- Put the wheat tortillas on a flat surface and distribute the

potato mixture on all the tortillas.
- Wrap them up and seal them with water.
- Heat the air fryer to 350 F. Put ½ tbsp. of coconut oil in it and place the burritos into it. Cook for 8-10 minutes.
- Serve and enjoy!

Nutritional Analysis (Per Serving)
Calories 393
Total fat 12.8g
Carbs 59.6g
Protein 11.1g

Air Fryer Yuca Fries

Tasty yuca fries seasoned with paprika, basil, and rosemary!

Serving Size: 4 persons

Prep Time: 10 minutes

Cooking Time: 25 minutes

Ingredients Needed

- 2 large yuccas
- 1 sprig of basil
- 1 sprig of rosemary
- 1 tablespoon of paprika
- 1 tablespoon of coconut oil
- ½ teaspoon of sea salt
- ½ teaspoon of pepper

Method of Preparation

- Cut the yuccas into juliennes. Put them into a bowl with water to prevent them from turning black.
- Thinly chop rosemary and basil.
- Mix the chopped leaves with the paprika, salt, and pepper.
- Remove the yuca from the water and coat them with the previous mixture.
- Heat air fryer to 350 F. and add the coconut oil.
- Place the yuca slices into the fryer and cook for 25 minutes until golden.
- Serve and enjoy!

Nutritional Analysis (Per Serving)

Calories 156

Total fat 3.7g

Carbs 28.3g
Protein 3.3g

Coconut Artichoke Fries

Delicious artichoke hearts breaded with almond and coconut

Serving Size: 4 persons

Prep Time: 15 minutes

Cooking Time: 30 minutes

Ingredients Needed

- 2 cloves of garlic
- 1 cup of almond flour
- 1 teaspoon of salt
- ½ teaspoon of black pepper
- 2 pounds of artichoke hearts
- 1 cup of shredded coconut
- 1 tablespoon of coconut oil

Method of Preparation

- Drain the artichokes and cut them into medium squares. Set aside.
- In a food processor, blend the garlic with the coconut for 1 minute. Stir in the salt and pepper.
- Mix the almond flour with the previous mixture.
- Heat air fryer to 375 F and add the coconut oil.
- Coat the artichoke hearts with coconut mixture and place them into the fryer. Cook for 12 minutes.
- Serve and enjoy!

Nutritional Analysis (Per Serving)

Calories 310

Total fat 19.2g

Carbs 31.3g

Protein 12g

Parmesan Eggplant

Tasty eggplant slices topped with marinara sauce!

    Serving Size: 4 persons

    Prep Time: 15 minutes

    Cooking Time: 30 minutes

Ingredients Needed

- 1 large eggplant
- 1 cup of marinara sauce
- 2 tablespoon of olive oil
- 1 cup of walnuts
- 1 tablespoon of dried basil
- 1 tablespoon of dried rosemary
- Salt and pepper to taste

Method of Preparation

- Slice the eggplant into ½ inch slices. Set aside.
- In a food processor, blend the walnuts for about 10-15 seconds.
- Thinly chop the basil and the rosemary.
- Heat air fryer to 375 F.
- Oil each eggplant slice with olive oil and place them into the fryer.
- Top each slice with walnuts, marinara sauce, basil, and rosemary.
- Cook for 12 minutes. Add salt and pepper.
- Serve and enjoy!

Nutritional Analysis (Per Serving)

Calories 339

Total fat 27.5g

Carbs 19g
Protein 9.8g

Portobello Pizza

Delicious pizza bites with basil, tomato and pecan nuts!

Serving Size: 4 persons

Prep Time: 15 minutes

Cooking Time: 30 minutes

Ingredients Needed

- 4 large Portobello mushrooms
- 3 cloves of garlic
- 1 sprig of basil
- ½ red onion
- 2 tablespoon olive oil
- ½ cup of cherry tomatoes
- ½ cup of pecan nuts
- Salt and pepper to taste

Method of Preparation

- Remove the stems and the gills from the mushrooms.
- Thinly chop the garlic cloves.
- Chop the basil.
- Slice the red onion.
- Slice the cherry tomatoes.
- In a food processor, blend the pecan nuts for 10 seconds.
- Top each mushroom with pecan nuts, tomato slices, onion slices, basil, and garlic (in that order).
- Heat air fryer to 375 F and add the oil in it.
- Place each Portobello pizza into the fryer and cook 15 minutes. Season with salt and pepper.
- Serve and enjoy!

Nutritional Analysis (Per Serving)
Calories 311
Total fat 29.4g
Carbs 10.4g
Protein 6.9g

Air Fryer Onion Rings

Crunchy and healthy onion rings breaded with almond flour!

Serving Size: 4 persons

Prep Time: 15 minutes

Cooking Time: 30 minutes

Ingredients Needed

2 large onions

½ cup of almond flour

1 tablespoon of complete seasoning

½ cup of coconut cream

1 tablespoon of dried basil

1 tablespoon of dried oregano

½ teaspoon of salt

½ teaspoon of pepper

1 tablespoon of coconut oil

1 cup of Prego sauce

Method of Preparation

- Slice the onions into ½ inch slices.
- Separate all the onion slices and put them aside.
- In a food processor, blend the basil, oregano, salt, and pepper.
- Mix the almond flour with complete seasoning and the previous mixture.
- Stir in the coconut cream and mix well until fully combined.
- Heat air fryer to 375 F and add the coconut oil.
- Deep each onion ring into the almond mixture and place them into the fryer.
- Cook for 12-15 minutes.
- Serve onion rings and accompany with Prego sauce. Enjoy!

Nutritional Analysis (Per Serving)

Calories 127
Total fat 9.1g
Carbs 10.8g
Protein 2.5g

Air Fryer Buffalo Cauliflower

Crunchy and spicy cauliflower florets seasoned with chili powder and garlic!

Serving Size: 4 persons
Prep Time: 10 minutes
Cooking Time: 25 minutes

Ingredients Needed

- 1 large cauliflower
- ½ cup of coconut oil
- ½ cup of tabasco spicy sauce
- 1 teaspoon of pepper
- 1 teaspoon of salt
- 1 teaspoon of chili powder
- 1 teaspoon of paprika
- 4 cloves of garlic
- ⅛ cup of flour
- ⅛ cup of shredded coconut
- ⅛ cup of almond milk
- 1 tablespoon of olive oil

Method of Preparation

- Cut the cauliflower into medium florets. Place the in a bowl, and set aside.
- Thinly slice the garlic.
- Heat a stove over medium heat and add the spicy sauce, pepper, salt, chili powder, paprika, garlic, and coconut oil. Heat for five minutes, stirring constantly. Set aside.
- In a bowl, mix the coconut, flour, and almond milk.
- Coat the cauliflower florets with the previous mixture.

- Heat air fryer to 375 F and add the olive oil into it.
- Place cauliflower florets into the fryer and cook for 12-15 minutes.
- Serve on a large bowl and pour the spicy sauce over them, Enjoy!

Nutritional Analysis (Per Serving)
Calories 372
Total fat 32.1g
Carbs 20g
Protein 7g

Roasted Brussel Sprouts

An easy and simple recipe to enjoy! Brussel sprouts seasoned with cumin and oregano!

Serving Size: 4 persons

Prep Time: 5 minutes

Cooking Time: 20 minutes

Ingredients Needed

- 1 pound of Brussel sprouts
- ⅛ cup of slivered almonds
- 1 tablespoon of coconut oil
- 1 teaspoon of cumin
- 1 teaspoon of dried oregano
- ⅛ cup of soy sauce
- 1 teaspoon of Himalayan salt
- 1 teaspoon of pepper

Method of Preparation

- Heat an air fryer to 375 F.
- In a large bowl, place the Brussel sprouts and add the cumin, oregano, soy sauce, salt, pepper, and almonds. Combine well.
- Put the coconut oil in the fryer.
- Add the Brussels sprouts into the fryer and let them cook for 18-20 minutes.
- Serve and enjoy!

Nutritional Analysis (Per Serving)

Calories 127

Total fat 7.5g

Carbs 12.9g

Protein 5.8g

Fried Mushrooms

Amazing breaded mushrooms with the unique flavor of basil!
Serving Size: 4 persons
Prep Time: 5 minutes
Cooking Time: 20 minutes
Ingredients Needed

- 1 pound of mushrooms
- ½ cup of almond flour
- 1 cup of almond milk
- ¼ cup of dried basil leaves
- 4 cloves of garlic
- ¼ of an onion
- 1 sprig of thyme
- 1 tablespoon of coconut oil
- 1 teaspoon of sea salt
- 1 teaspoon of pepper
- ½ cup of Caesar dressing

Method of Preparation

- Thinly chop the basil, garlic, onion, and thyme.
- Mix the almond flour with the chopped ingredients and the salt and pepper.
- Mix the previous mixture with the almond milk and combine well until you have a thick consistency.
- Deep all the mushrooms into the previous mixture and place them in a bowl.
- Heat air fryer to 375 F and add the coconut oil.
- Put all of the mushrooms into the fryer and cook for 15-20 minutes.

- Serve with dressing and enjoy!

Nutritional Analysis (Per Serving)
Calories 346
Total fat 29.2g
Carbs 19.6g
Protein 8.7g

Stuffed Air Fryer Potatoes

Delicious baked potato stuffed with spinach and mushrooms!

Serving Size: 4 persons

Prep Time: 10 minutes

Cooking Time: 25 minutes

Ingredients Needed

- 2 large potatoes
- 1 cup of sliced mushrooms
- 1 tablespoon of coconut oil
- 1 tablespoon of thyme
- 1 tablespoon of basil
- ⅛ cup of coconut milk
- 1 cup of spinach leaves

Method of Preparation

- Boil the potatoes on a pot with 1 liter of water for 5 minutes until soft.
- In a pan, sauté the mushrooms and the spinach with the coconut oil.
- Add the coconut milk and continue cooking for 2 more minutes. Set aside.
- Thinly chop the basil and thyme.
- Heat air fryer to 375 F.
- Stuff each potato with the mushrooms mixture and top with the basil and thyme.
- Place the stuffed potatoes into the fryer and cook for 20 minutes.
- Serve and enjoy!

Nutritional Analysis (Per Serving)
Calories 164
Total fat 3.7g
Carbs 30.3g
Protein 3.9g

Black Beans Morning Wrap

A delicious wrap made of black beans, avocado, and cilantro!

Serving Size: 4 persons

Prep Time: 10 minutes

Cooking Time: 25 minutes

Ingredients Needed

- 4 medium wheat tortillas
- 1 large avocado
- 1 cup of black beans, cooked
- 1 tablespoon of coconut oil
- ½ cup of cilantro leaves
- 1 jalapeno pepper
- 1 teaspoon of sea salt
- 1 teaspoon of white pepper
- 2 cloves of garlic
- ¼ cup of Prego sauce

Method of Preparation

- Cut the avocado in half, remove the seed and slice the avocado.
- Thinly chop the garlic cloves, jalapeno and cilantro leaves.
- Heat a pan with coconut oil and cook the garlic for 30 seconds, then add the cilantro, black beans, salt, pepper, jalapeno, and Prego sauce. Place this mixture in a bowl and set aside.
- Put the tortillas on a flat surface and distribute the avocado slices and beans mixture on each tortilla.
- Wrap the tortillas and seal with water.
- Heat air fryer to 375 F.
- Place the wraps into the fryer and cook for 15 minutes.
- Serve and enjoy!

Nutritional Analysis (Per Serving)
Calories 387
Total fat 16.1g
Carbs 48.5g
Protein 14.8g

Fried Cucumbers

Delicious breaded cucumbers, seasoned with cumin, mint, and garlic!
Serving Size: 4 persons
Prep Time: 10 minutes
Cooking Time: 15 minutes
Ingredients Needed

- 2 large cucumbers
- 1 cup of almond flour
- 1 tablespoon of cumin
- ¼ cup of mint leaves
- 4 cloves of garlic
- 1 teaspoon of Himalayan salt
- 1 teaspoon of pepper
- 1 cup of coconut cream
- 1 tablespoon of coconut oil

Method of Preparation

- In a food processor, blend the cumin, mint, and garlic for 1 minute or until thinly chopped.
- Mix the combines leaves with the almond flour, salt, and pepper. Put this mixture in a bowl.
- Slice the cucumbers into ½ inch slices.
- Heat air fryer to 375 F and the coconut oil into it.
- Deep each cucumber slice into the coconut milk and then pass them through the flour mixture.
- Place cucumber slices into the fryer and cook for 15 minutes.
- Serve and enjoy!

Nutritional Analysis (Per Serving)

Calories 304
Total fat 27g
Carbs 15g
Protein 6.8g

Air Fried Apples

Sweet and tasty apples stuffed with almonds and raisins

Serving Size: 4 persons

Prep Time: 10 minutes

Cooking Time: 20 minutes

Ingredients Needed

- 4 apples
- ½ cup of sliced almonds
- ½ cup of raisins
- ½ cup of raw honey

Method of Preparation

- Heat air fryer to 375 F.
- Remove the core from the apples.
- In a bowl, mix the almonds, raisings, and honey.
- Stuff each apple in the whole where the cores were removed.
- Place stuffed apples into the fryer and cook for 20 minutes.
- Serve and enjoy!

Nutritional Analysis (Per Serving)

Calories 368

Total fat 6.4g

Carbs 82.6g

Protein 3.8g

Apple Cinnamon Chips

Delicious apple chips topped with mint and cinnamon!

Serving Size: 4 persons

Prep Time: 5 minutes

Cooking Time: 25 minutes

Ingredients Needed

- 4 green apples
- 1 tablespoon of mint leaves
- 1 tablespoon of cinnamon powder
- 1 tablespoon of grated coconut
- 1 tablespoon of coconut oil

Method of Preparation

- Heat air fryer to 250 F.
- Thinly slice the apples.
- Thinly chop the mint.
- Coat the apple chips with the coconut oil.
- Place apple chips into the fryer.
- Pour the mint, coconut, and cinnamon over the chips and cook for 25 minutes.
- Serve and enjoy!

Nutritional Analysis (Per Serving)

Calories 150

Total fat 4.2g

Carbs 31.2g

Protein 0.7g

Tangerine Coconut Fries

Sweet and citric tangerine slices fried with coconut!

Serving Size: 4 persons

Prep Time: 5 minutes

Cooking Time: 25 minutes

Ingredients Needed

- 4 tangerines
- 1 cup of grated coconut
- 2 tablespoon of raw honey
- 1 tablespoon of lemon juice
- ¼ cups of cashews

Method of Preparation

- Heat air fryer to 375 F.
- Mix the honey with the lemon juice.
- Separate the supremes from the tangerines and set aside.
- Coat the supremes with the raw honey and then pass them through the coconut.
- Place the tangerines into the fryer and cook for 20-25 minutes.
- Serve with cashews, enjoy!

Nutritional Analysis (Per Serving)

Calories 197

Total fat 10.9g

Carbs 25.8g

Protein 2.7g

Banana Boats

Delicious bananas topped with coconut, chocolate, and almonds!
Serving Size: 4 persons
Prep Time: 5 minutes
Cooking Time: 15 minutes
Ingredients Needed

- 4 large bananas
- ¼ cup of chocolate chips
- ¼ of sliced almonds
- ½ cup of grated coconut
- 1 tablespoon of coconut oil
- 2 tablespoons of raw honey

Method of Preparation

- Heat air fryer to 375 F.
- With a knife, cut the bananas lengthwise until the middle of them.
- Top each banana with almonds, coconut and chocolate chips.
- Place banana boats into the fryer and cook for 15 minutes.
- Serve and enjoy!

Nutritional Analysis (Per Serving)
Calories 274
Total fat 10.3g
Carbs 47.5g
Protein 2.7g

Air Fried Yellow Corn

Delicious corn seasoned with garlic, oregano, and basil!

Serving Size: 4 persons

Prep Time: 5 minutes

Cooking Time: 25 minutes

Ingredients Needed

- 4 sweet yellow corn
- 1 tablespoon of dried oregano
- 1 tablespoon of dried basil
- 4 cloves of garlic
- 2 tablespoon of coconut oil
- 1 teaspoon of sea salt
- 1 teaspoon of white pepper

Method of Preparation

- Heat air fryer to 375 F.
- Thinly chop the oregano basil and garlic.
- Mix the chopped ingredients with the coconut oil, salt, and pepper.
- Coat each corn with the previous mixture,
- Place the corn into the fryer and cook for 25 minutes.
- Serve and enjoy!

Nutritional Analysis (Per Serving)

Calories 200

Total fat 8.8g

Carbs 31.1g

Protein 5.4g

Carrot Fries for Breakfast

Sweet and crunchy carrot French fries accompanied with chickpeas!
Serving Size: 4 persons
Prep Time: 10 minutes
Cooking Time: 15 minutes
Ingredients Needed

- 2 large carrots
- 2 cups of chickpeas, soaked
- 4 cloves of garlic
- ½ onion
- 1 tablespoon of thyme leaves
- 1 teaspoon of complete seasoning
- ½ teaspoon of salt
- ½ teaspoon of pepper
- 1 tablespoon of coconut oil

Method of Preparation

- Heat air fryer to 375 F.
- Cut the carrots into juliennes.
- Thinly chop the garlic, thyme, and onion.
- Heat a pan with ½ tablespoon of coconut oil and cook the chopped onion until it's transparent, then add the chickpeas and cook for 3 more minutes. Set aside.
- Coat the carrot pieces with coconut oil and top them with garlic and thyme.
- Place carrot fries into the fryer and cook for 15 minutes. Season with salt and pepper to taste.
- Serve with chickpeas, enjoy!

Nutritional Analysis (Per Serving)

Calories 421

Total fat 9.5g

Carbs 67.1g

Protein 20 g

Air Fried Spicy Burrito

Amazing burrito stuffed with black beans, chickpeas, and lettuce!
Serving Size: 4 persons
Prep Time: 10 minutes
Cooking Time: 15 minutes
Ingredients Needed

- 4 large wheat tortillas
- 1 cup of black beans, cooked
- 1 cup of chickpeas, cooked
- 1 head of lettuce
- 4 cloves of garlic
- ½ onion
- 1 teaspoon of pepper
- ¼ cup of chipotle sauce
- 1 teaspoon of sea salt
- 1 tablespoon of coconut oil

Method of Preparation

- Heat air fryer to 375 F.
- Thinly chop the lettuce and set aside.
- Thinly chop the garlic cloves and the onion.
- Heat a pan with coconut oil and cook the onion and garlic until the onion becomes transparent. Add the black beans and chickpeas and cook for 4 more minutes.
- Place the tortillas on a flat surface and distribute the lettuce and the beans mixture on each tortilla, and top with chipotle sauce. Wrap the tortillas and seal them with water.
- Place the burritos into the fryer and cook for 15 minutes.
- Serve and enjoy!

Nutritional Analysis (Per Serving)

Calories 494

Total fat 9.3g

Carbs 80.6g

Protein 23.9g

Asparagus Stuffed Potatoes

Stuffed mashed potatoes with the unique flavor of asparagus!
Serving Size: 4 persons
Prep Time: 15 minutes
Cooking Time: 20 minutes
Ingredients Needed

- 1 handful of asparagus
- 3 large potatoes
- 5 cloves of garlic
- ½ red onion
- 1 teaspoon of sea salt
- 1 teaspoon of pepper
- ¼ cup of coconut cream
- 1 tablespoon of coconut oil
- 1 cup of spinach leaves

Method of Preparation

- Peel the potatoes and boil them on a pot with 1 liter of water. Boil for 10 minutes until soft.
- Thinly chop the garlic, onion, asparagus, and spinach.
- Heat a stove with coconut oil and cook the chopped ingredients for 4 minutes and set aside.
- Mash the potatoes and mix with the coconut cream. Season with salt and pepper.
- Form medium balls with the mashed potatoes and stuff them with the asparagus mixture. Put them in a large bowl and cover them with plastic wrap. Refrigerate for 30 min.
- Heat air fryer to 400 F.
- Place stuffed potatoes into the fryer and cook for 20 minutes

until browned.
- Serve and enjoy!

Nutritional Analysis (Per Serving)
Calories 274
Total fat 7.4g
Carbs 48.4g
Protein 6.2g

Air Fried Zucchini Chips

Tasty zucchini chips bread with coconut and seasoned with peppermint!
Serving Size: 4 persons
Prep Time: 15 minutes
Cooking Time: 25 minutes

Ingredients Needed

- 2 large zucchinis
- 1 cup of grated coconut
- ½ cup of peppermint leaves
- 1 teaspoon of salt
- 1 teaspoon of pepper
- 1 cup of almond milk
- 1 tablespoon of olive oil

Method of Preparation

- Thinly slice the zucchinis.
- Thinly chop the peppermint.
- Mix the coconut with the peppermint, salt, and pepper.
- Deep each zucchini slice into the milk and pass them through the coconut.
- Heat the air fryer to 375 F and add the olive oil.
- Place the zucchini slices into the fryer and cook for 12-15 minutes.
- Serve and enjoy!

Nutritional Analysis (Per Serving)
Calories 271
Total fat 24.9g
Carbs 13.1g

Protein 4.4g

9 781386 342496